POCKET GUIDES
FOR NURSING AND HEALTH CARE

MULTIDISCIPLINARY WORKING

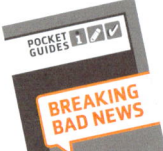
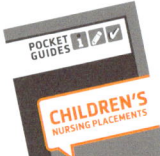
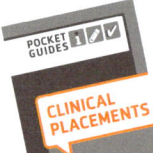
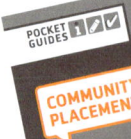

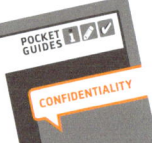

A unique series of pocket-sized books designed to help healthcare students

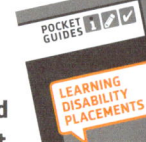

"All the information was clear and concise, this book is exactly what I was looking for." ★★★★★

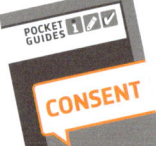

"A great little guide. All the basic information needed to have a quick reference." ★★★★★

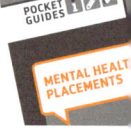

"A very useful, well-written and practical pocket book." ★★★★★

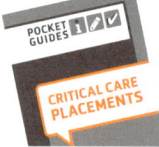

"Written by students for students. A must for any student about to head on placement."
★★★★

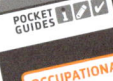
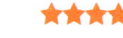
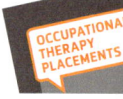

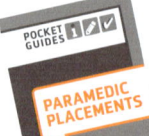
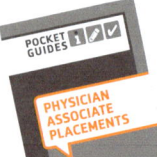
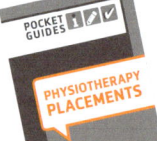
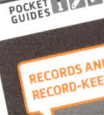

POCKET GUIDES
FOR NURSING AND HEALTH CARE

MULTIDISCIPLINARY WORKING

Edited by
Sam Humphrey and Pippa Chillman
De Montfort University
Leicester

Lantern

© Lantern Publishing Ltd, 2025
ISBN 9781914962288

First published 2025

All rights, including for text and data mining (TDM), artificial intelligence (AI) training, and similar technologies, are reserved. No part of this book may be reproduced or transmitted, in any form or by any means, without permission.

A CIP catalogue record for this book is available from the British Library.

Lantern Publishing Limited, The Old Hayloft, Vantage Business Park, Bloxham Road, Banbury OX16 9UX, UK
www.lanternpublishing.com

The authors and publisher have made every attempt to ensure the content of this book is up to date and accurate. However, healthcare knowledge and information is changing all the time so the reader is advised to double-check any information in this text on drug usage, treatment procedures, the use of equipment, etc. to confirm that it complies with the latest safety recommendations, standards of practice and legislation, as well as local Trust policies and procedures. Students are advised to check with their tutor and/or practice supervisor before carrying out any of the procedures in this textbook.

Typeset by Medlar Publishing Solutions Pvt Ltd, India
Printed and bound in the UK

Last digit is the print number: 10 9 8 7 6 5 4 3 2 1

Contents

Preface ix
Acknowledgements x
List of contributors xi
Abbreviations xiv

Preparing for multidisciplinary team (MDT) working

1. Introducing multidisciplinary working 2
2. The MDT and professions 'grab-sheet' 3
3. Nursing fields and common nursing roles 10
    3.1 Adult nursing 11
    3.2 Children's nursing 12
    3.3 Mental Health nursing 13
    3.4 Learning Disability nursing 14
4. Allied Health Professionals 15
    4.1 How AHPs contribute to the MDT 15
    4.2 Learning more about AHPs 16
5. Social care professions 17
    5.1 The role of social care and its links with other professions 17
    5.2 The biopsychosocial model in social care 19
6. Common situations requiring MDT input 21
    6.1 Example A: Emergency and trauma 21
    6.2 Example B: Mental health 22
    6.3 Example C: Obstetric emergency 23
    6.4 Example D: Disability and rehabilitation 24
7. Student roles within the MDT 26
    7.1 Getting involved 26
    7.2 Expectations for students in the MDT 26

	7.3	Benefits of involvement 27
	7.4	Involvement challenges (and solutions)...... 28
	7.5	Practical tips 29
8.	Building confidence.......................... 30	
	8.1	Speaking up 30
	8.2	Reflecting on mistakes 31
	8.3	Supporting patients to be confident 31
	8.4	Ways to build confidence 32

Collaborative working within the MDT

9.	Integrating into teams...................... 36	
	9.1	What are the benefits to staff and patient care?...................... 36
	9.2	Potential difficulties of integrating when you are 'the student'.................... 38
10.	Communication strategies to support integration.. 39	
	10.1	SBAR................................... 39
	10.2	Demonstrating active listening and assertiveness 40
	10.3	Understanding hierarchies and overcoming communication barriers to build relationships 42
11.	Civility..................................... 44	
	11.1	The Civility Saves Lives campaign 45
	11.2	Acting on civility 46
12.	Inclusivity and teamwork within care 48	
	12.1	Key principles of inclusivity and teamwork... 48
	12.2	Benefits of inclusivity and teamwork........ 49
	12.3	Challenges facing inclusivity and teamwork .. 49
	12.4	Building an inclusive team environment 50

13. Managing differing priorities and
potential conflict 52
    13.1 Balancing urgent and non-urgent needs 52
    13.2 Managing differing priorities in an MDT 54
    13.3 Potential conflict in MDTs 55
14. Use of language 57
    14.1 Common language barriers in MDTs 57
    14.2 Strategies for clear communication
and language 58
15. MDT working: Good practice advice 59

Enhancing the MDT experience

16. Professional identity 64
    16.1 The role of professional identity
in MDT working 65
    16.2 Strengthening professional identity
in MDTs 65
17. Collaboration with stakeholders 67
    17.1 Key principles of collaboration
with stakeholders 67
18. Co-production with patients / service users 70
    18.1 Core principles of co-production 70
19. Patient safety 73
    19.1 The role of the MDT in patient safety 74
    19.2 Strategies for enhancing patient safety 75
20. Professional development opportunities 78
    20.1 Types of professional development
opportunities for MDT members 79
    20.2 How to get started with professional
development in an MDT 80

21. Scenarios for guided reflection and action planning 81
    21.1 Common scenarios...................... 82
22. Further understanding: ethics and integrity in MDT working 86
23. The importance of self-care for health and social care professionals working within the MDT.................................... 90

Preface

This pocket guide to multidisciplinary working is aimed at nursing, allied health and social care students and is an accessible introductory text for students seeking to develop their teamworking skills.

Offering insight regarding the dynamic landscape of modern health and social care, this book will help you to understand the principles of collaboration and teamwork, essential for providing effective patient-centred care within a multidisciplinary team (MDT).

Within these pages, you will learn:

- the core principles of understanding multidisciplinary working, emphasising person-centred care, student roles within the MDT and why different perspectives are vital to enhance patient experience
- about the importance of civility and inclusivity towards each other
- about the complexity of managing differing priorities, potential conflicts between professionals and communication strategies
- real scenarios: the opportunity to read case studies, showcasing the challenges and benefits of MDT working
- career development: consider how effective MDT working not only benefits patients but also boosts professional growth and development
- practical tools: access valuable tools, strategies and tips to enhance your ability to collaborate effectively with diverse teams of health and social care professionals.

Most importantly, this book has been written primarily *by* students, *for* students. Student volunteers from the Council of Deans' #150Leaders programme from a wide variety of disciplines have written about the areas of multidisciplinary working that matter to them.

This pocket guide is a compact and helpful guide for student health, allied and social care professionals working within dynamic health and social care teams, equipping you with the knowledge and skills required to be an effective multidisciplinary team member.

Sam Humphrey
Pippa Chillman

Acknowledgements

We would like to thank the Council of Deans for supporting the project and the student volunteers on the #150Leaders programme for all of their hard work and contributions to this pocket guide.

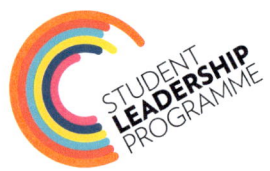

List of contributors

George Bowles
Student Paramedic, Oxford Brookes University
- *Sections contributed to: 17, 19, 21 and 22*

Lily Carline
Healthcare Science (Cardiac Physiology), BSc (Hons), Swansea University
- *Sections contributed to: 11 and 20*

Lauren Caulfield
Student Midwife, University of Manchester
- *Sections contributed to: 7, 9, 10 and 17*

Pippa Chillman
Senior Lecturer in Mental Health Nursing and Mental Health Nursing Field Lead, De Montfort University, Leicester
- *Sections contributed to: 5, 14, 16, 22 and 23*

Minne Christensen
Student Learning Disability Nurse, Edinburgh Napier University
- *Sections contributed to: 1, 7 and 8*

Dean Cox
Student Community Mental Health Occupational Therapy Apprentice, University of Hertfordshire
- *Sections contributed to: 4, 6, 8 and 12*

Harris Cunningham

Student Paramedic, Queen Margaret University

- *Sections contributed to: 6, 8, 15* and *22*

Francesca Dixon

Student Radiographer, Keele University

- *Sections contributed to: 7, 12* and *18*

Bronwyn Flower-Bond

Student Adult Nurse, University of Winchester

- *Sections contributed to: 3, 15, 18* and *22*

Ella Foster

Student Adult and Mental Health Nurse, University of Leicester

- *Sections contributed to: 2, 3* and *9*

Sarah Louise Hough

Student Learning Disability Nurse, University of the West of England

- *Sections contributed to: 3, 12, 15* and *22*

Sam Humphrey

Senior Lecturer in Learning Disability Nursing and Programme Leader; BSc (Hons) Nursing (with NMC registration), De Montfort University, Leicester

- *Sections contributed to: 5, 14, 16, 22* and *23*

Leanne Milne

Student Midwife, University of the West of Scotland

- *Sections contributed to:* 6 and 11

Divanshi Sharma

Student Adult Nurse, University of Roehampton London

- *Sections contributed to:* 7 and 19

Jake Shaw

Student Mental Health Nurse, University of Worcester

- *Sections contributed to:* 1, 6, 10 and 19

Kit Sinclair

Student Speech and Language Therapist, City University, London

- *Sections contributed to:* 4, 6, 11 and 20

Amelia Surrey

Student Therapeutic Radiographer, Health Sciences University

- *Sections contributed to:* 4, 8, 9 and 13

Thalia Tzing Lam Lau

Student Physiotherapist, Cardiff University

- *Sections contributed to:* 2, 9, 21 and 22

Abbreviations

AHP	Allied Health Professional
CDSS	clinical decision support systems
CEN	Clinical Excellence Network
CPD	continuing professional development
CQC	Care Quality Commission
EHR	electronic health record
GP	general practice/practitioner
HCPC	Health and Care Professions Council
IPE	Interprofessional education
MDT	multidisciplinary team
MRSA	methicillin-resistant *Staphylococcus aureus*
NEWS	National Early Warning Score
RCA	root cause analysis
SBAR	Situation, Background, Assessment, Recommendation
SMART	Specific, Measurable, Achievable, Relevant and Time-bound
TAG	Threshold Assessment Grid

> Confusion in the use of abbreviations has been cited as the reason for some clinical incidents. Therefore you should use these abbreviations with caution and only in line with local Trusts' Clinical Governance recommendations which vary between departments!

Add your own abbreviations here:

Preparing for multidisciplinary team (MDT) working

1. Introducing multidisciplinary working 2
2. The MDT and professions 'grab-sheet' 3
3. Nursing fields and common nursing roles 10
4. Allied Health Professionals 15
5. Social care professions 17
6. Common situations requiring MDT input 21
7. Student roles within the MDT 26
8. Building confidence 30

1. Introducing multidisciplinary working

In multidisciplinary team (MDT) working, each member has a distinct role.

An MDT consists of professionals and team members from various specialities working together to deliver holistic, person-centred care to people from across the lifespan.

In the sections that follow, common members of the MDT will be explored:

- Nursing – *Section 3*
- Allied Health Professionals – *Section 4*
- Social care professions – *Section 5*

Then ways to explore your preparation for MDT working will be discussed:

- Examples of common situations requiring MDT input – *Section 6*
- Student roles within the MDT – *Section 7*
- Building confidence – *Section 8*

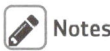 Notes

The MDT and professions 'grab-sheet'

2

As a student health and social care worker, you'll work with a range of professionals who are part of a multidisciplinary team (MDT). The MDT describes a group of individuals with unique professions that allow them to work together in planning and providing the best treatment and care to patients.

Here are some examples of professionals you may work alongside, with space to add others you encounter:

Nursing and Midwifery	
Nurses and Midwives deliver and coordinate patient-centred care, addressing physical, emotional and social needs that individuals may struggle to manage on their own. Nursing practice includes four main fields, along with the role of Nursing Associate, each contributing to holistic care.	
Adult Nurse	Generally provides care for people above the age of 18
Children's / Paediatric Nurse	Generally provides care for people from birth to the age of 18
Mental Health Nurse	Provides support for people of all ages, focusing on psychiatric health
Learning Disability Nurse	Provides support for people of all ages who require specialised provision for a learning disability
Nursing Associate	Provides direct patient care, supporting registered nurses by monitoring patient conditions and carrying out clinical tasks

Nursing and Midwifery	
Midwife	Supports and cares for women, their babies and families throughout all stages of pregnancy and childbirth
Dual Registrant	Registered in two parts of the NMC register (e.g. Learning Disability and Mental Health Nursing, or Adult Nursing and Midwifery) and can practise in either field

Medics	
Anaesthesiologist	Administers anaesthesia and monitors patients' vital signs before, during and after surgery; they focus on safety, comfort and pain management
Doctor	Diagnoses, treats and prevents disease and injuries, ensuring physical and mental wellbeing through holistic care
Psychiatrist	A medical doctor who diagnoses, treats and helps manage mental health conditions through therapy, medication and other interventions
Surgeon	Specialising in performing operative procedures, they are trained in diagnosing conditions, and planning and performing surgeries, alongside managing post-operative recovery

Allied Health Professionals (AHPs)

AHPs work with patients in a range of specialities, using their expertise to assess, treat and support individuals across a range of health conditions. Each AHP role contributes to rehabilitation, recovery and overall wellbeing through a holistic, patient-centred approach. Working across various settings, AHPs collaborate within MDTs to improve health outcomes and enhance quality of life.

Art therapist	Art therapists use creative expression to help individuals process and manage confusing or distressing emotions
Dietitian	Uses nutritional research to promote healthy eating and prevent diseases such as obesity and malnutrition, while developing nutrition support plans and dietary interventions to enhance patient care
Drama therapist	Uses role play, voice work, movement and storytelling to help individuals explore and address personal and social challenges
Music therapist	Uses music to help individuals express and process emotions that are difficult to verbalise
Occupational Therapist	Focuses on functional everyday living such as dressing, bathing and cooking Aims to improve patients' quality of life to allow them to live as independently as possible
Operating Department Practitioner	A healthcare professional who supports surgical teams during operations, ensuring patient safety, managing anaesthesia and assisting with recovery
Orthoptist	A field for diagnosing and treating visual disorders related to eye movement and coordination, often using therapies to correct these

Allied Health Professionals (AHPs)	
Osteopath	Specialises in the musculoskeletal system, using movement, stretching and massage to detect, treat and prevent health issues
Paramedic	Provides emergency care to patients, stabilising them in pre-hospital settings such as accident scenes or transportation to a medical facility
Physiotherapist	Works to rehabilitate patients in diagnosis and treatment of illnesses Creates tailored treatment plans for recovery from injuries, surgeries or illnesses limiting movement and physical function
Podiatrist	Provides treatment and care for individuals with foot and lower limb conditions resulting from injury or illness
Prosthetist and orthotist	Prosthetists assess, design and provide prosthetic limbs to enhance the lives of individuals Orthotists prescribe, design and supply orthoses to support and protect the neuromuscular and skeletal systems
Radiographer	Works either *diagnostically*, using medical imaging (such as X-rays or CT scans) to aid in diagnosing an injury or illness, or *therapeutically*, delivering radiation treatment for cancer and supporting patients through this treatment pathway
Speech and Language Therapist	Provides treatment and support for patients who have communication, language and swallowing difficulties

Social care roles	
Activities worker	Plans and facilitates social activities, outings and entertainment for individuals needing care and support, encouraging their participation
Advocacy worker	Helps vulnerable individuals express their views and ensures their best interests are considered in decisions affecting their lives
Personal assistant	Assists individuals in maintaining maximum independence, typically within their own home or community
Social worker	Works mostly with vulnerable people to solve problems, meet needs and improve life quality

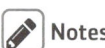 Notes

Additional roles	
Healthcare Assistant	Assists clinical staff in giving person-centred care to patients; achieved through tasks such as monitoring vitals, maintaining hygiene, ensuring comfort and feeding
Pharmacist	Focuses on drug information and prescribing, whilst also troubleshooting any related pharmaceutical care issues
Psychologist	Uses expertise, risk assessment and management to offer a psychological perspective to mental state; this develops a shared understanding between professionals and patients

Notes

3. Nursing fields and common nursing roles

There are four main registered nursing fields: Adult, Children's (sometimes referred to as Children and Adolescent, or Paediatric nursing), Mental Health, and Learning Disability. All fields can work in different types of areas such as hospitals, community healthcare centres, outpatient clinics, specialist units, secure residential units and patients' homes. All fields of nursing deliver holistic and person-centred care.

Below are some examples of specialist roles within each field which you may find within a team or MDT environment. There is space for you to add your own too. It is important to note that these fields can overlap; for example, transitions from childhood to adulthood when specialising in Learning Disability, and Autism in a Forensic Unit.

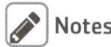 Notes

3.1 Adult nursing

Role	Description
Community Nurse	Provides care to patients away from clinical settings, often visiting people in their houses or residential homes
General Practice Nurse	Provides a range of primary health care within a GP surgery, such as vaccinating and wound care
Prison Nurse	Provides primary care for offenders; duties include emergency response, medicating and long-term condition management
Ward-based Staff Nurse	Treats patients in hospitals within a range of specialities, such as oncology and neurology

Notes

3.2 Children's nursing

Role	Description
Health Visitor	A specialist public health nurse who supports families with children under 5 years, providing health advice, developmental assessments, and safeguarding involvement alongside early interventions to promote wellbeing
NICU Nurse	Works within a hospital neonatal intensive care unit caring for newborns and premature infants
Paediatric Registered Nurse	Has understanding of child growth and development, and knows how to treat diseases and conditions in children
School Nurse	Works within a school with children and their families to reduce inequalities and promote public health, good health and wellbeing

 Notes

3.3 Mental Health nursing

Role	Description
Forensic Nurse	Manages and treats those within the criminal justice system, including those who encounter the criminal justice system because of their mental health or subsequent illness
	Centred around the assessment and management of risk posed by offenders; support can include at point of arrest, custody, in court, probation services or within prisons or in secure hospitals where offenders may serve out a conviction
Mental Health Liaison Nurse	Working within a primary care setting, a specialist mental health team who are able to support physical health staff with a person's mental health needs
	They can gather and share information between services and assess a patient, escalating needs further if required
Mental Health Nurse	Makes therapeutic use of psychological and psychosocial skills and interventions to engage with an individual to aid in managing their mental health and wellbeing
	This can be within a team, either in a ward, the community or specialist mental health service; or on a 1:1 basis with individuals
Specialised Practitioner	There are many specialisms within mental health to train further in, such as: perinatal, children's and adolescent, older persons, drug, alcohol or addiction services and eating disorders

3.4 Learning Disability nursing

Role	Description
Behaviour Specialist Nurse	Uses their better understanding of expressive behaviours to improve quality of life; this may be by analysing behaviour by using ABC (antecedent, behaviour, consequence) charts, understanding communication needs or creating a PBS (positive behaviour support) plan
Epilepsy Nurse Specialist	Manages treatment for epilepsy including medication, diet, reviews, education and understanding triggers Although epilepsy is a separate condition, it is more common for those with a learning disability to have epilepsy than the general population
Residential Home Nurse	Works within a residential home providing extra support, over and above that provided by a support worker/carer, for those who need it This could involve developing, delivering and monitoring a care and support programme, administration of medication via mouth or PEG, and enabling people with learning disabilities to live a fulfilled life
Specialist Autism Practitioner	Although autism is different from the definition of a learning disability, Learning Disability nurses can be most suitable for this role, due to overlaps in skill sets such as making reasonable adjustments and understanding communication and sensory needs

4 Allied Health Professionals

Allied Health Professionals (AHPs) are a group of clinicians practising under a protected job title which is regulated by the Health and Care Professions Council (HCPC). There are fourteen distinct AHP professions; these are listed in *Section 2*.

The history of AHPs dates back to the 1940s, relating to a group of practitioners who were 'supplementary to medicine' but did not have professional status. It wasn't until the 1960s that they gained official status, as their professional identity developed independently enough of the medical profession to be considered 'allied to medicine'. For more about professional identity, see *Section 16*.

4.1 How AHPs contribute to the MDT

AHPs cover a huge variety of skills, knowledge and experiences. For the NHS to deliver its 'Long-term Plan', it must significantly increase the number of AHPs and understand their potential role.

One way of doing this is by switching to an MDT approach, which enables a mix of skills and roles to enhance the patient's experience and improve their health care.

In this approach, AHPs can help the team to offer a holistic assessment and treatment of the patient.

With the right support and qualifications, AHPs can be empowered to deliver interventions without the need for a registered clinician. This approach could be more cost-effective, but all professionals should be aware of the risk to governance, and ensure AHPs are acting within their competency with regular supervision to ensure they are supported.

4.2 Learning more about AHPs

There are a huge range of resources out there to help you learn more about the valuable role of AHPs and how they can best be utilised in your MDT.

> To make it easy for you to access them, we have shortened web links to this format – simply type these into any web browser and you'll go to the right page!

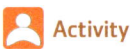 **Activity**

Why not start by watching the video at bit.ly/4iZHyDm? Meet Martha as she shares how various AHPs helped her during her mental health recovery journey.

Or, you could read the article at bit.ly/3YvicFT, which details a day in the life of a Paramedic First Contact Practitioner, a relatively new position which supports primary care practitioners in service of the NHS Long Term Plan's goal to deliver joined-up health care to patients.

Finally, keep an eye out for any continuing professional development (CPD) courses or days that your university, placement or employer may offer that give you the chance to meet and learn about AHPs relevant to your practice, and always make the most of any opportunity to work with them as part of an MDT.

5 Social care professions

Social care in the UK refers to a range of services designed to support individuals who need help due to age, disability, illness or other life circumstances.

It aims to promote wellbeing, independence and dignity, ensuring that people can lead fulfilling lives within their communities. Social care is primarily provided by local authorities, charities, private organisations and informal carers, such as family members and friends.

Unlike health care, which is generally free at the point of use under the NHS, many social care services are means-tested, meaning individuals may need to contribute to the cost of their care.

Social care encompasses various services, including residential care homes, domiciliary (home) care, day centres, respite care, and support for individuals with learning disabilities, mental health conditions and substance misuse issues.

It plays a crucial role in safeguarding vulnerable individuals, providing personal care, and facilitating access to resources that promote independence and inclusion.

5.1 The role of social care and its links with other professions

Social care does not operate in isolation; it is intrinsically linked with other professional fields, often through multidisciplinary working, to provide holistic support.

The collaboration between social care and other sectors is essential in addressing the complex needs of individuals. Some key professional links include the following:

- **Healthcare professionals:** social care often works closely with doctors, nurses, occupational therapists and physiotherapists, amongst others, to ensure that individuals receive comprehensive medical and rehabilitative support. For example, a person recovering from a stroke may require both home care assistance and physiotherapy to regain mobility.
- **Mental health services:** social workers, psychologists and community mental health nurses collaborate to support individuals with mental health conditions, ensuring they receive appropriate therapy, medication and social support to improve their quality of life.
- **Education and child services:** social care professionals, including social workers and family support workers, engage with schools and educational psychologists to support children with special educational needs, safeguarding concerns, or those in foster care.
- **Housing and welfare services:** social care professionals work alongside housing officers and benefits advisors to help individuals access suitable accommodation, financial assistance, and other essential resources that enable independent living.

Add any other social care collaboration examples you note as you work in MDTs:

- _____
- _____
- _____

5.2 The biopsychosocial model in social care

The biopsychosocial model (Engel, 1977) depicted in the figure below is an approach that considers biological, psychological and social factors when assessing and addressing an individual's needs. This model is particularly relevant in social care as it recognises the interconnected nature of health and wellbeing.

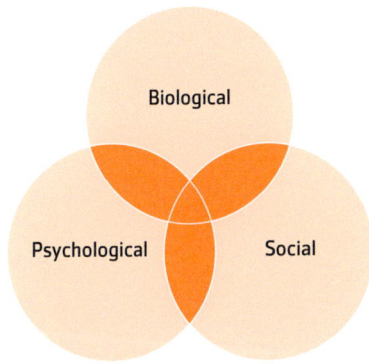

The Biopsychosocial Model (Engel, 1977).

- **Biological factors** include physical health conditions, disabilities, or age-related challenges that require medical and social care interventions.
- **Psychological factors** encompass mental health, emotional wellbeing, and cognitive conditions such as dementia, which necessitate therapeutic and supportive care.
- **Social factors** involve an individual's environment, relationships, financial status, and community engagement, all of which impact their overall wellbeing.

By adopting a biopsychosocial approach, social care professionals ensure that support is person-centred, addressing not just immediate needs but also long-term wellbeing. This holistic collaboration between social care and other professions is vital in creating a compassionate, effective support system for individuals and often forms a key part of their involvement within MDT situations.

Notes

Engel, G.L. (1977) The need for a new medical model: a challenge for biomedicine. *Science*, 196(4286): 129–136.

6 Common situations requiring MDT input

Below you will find some examples of common situations that will require MDT input to showcase the impact that each profession and professional has, on both the patient and the other professionals working within the MDT. Key professions within each example are highlighted in bold.

- Use these examples to consider if any situations you are seeing in your current placement may benefit from input from a wider MDT.
- There is space at the end of this section for you to record your own MDT situational example.
- You may wish to use these examples, or your own, to reflect on the roles and impact of MDT members as a way to check your understanding. For more about reflection and subsequent action planning, see *Section 21*.

6.1 Example A: Emergency and trauma

Paulina has been involved in a single-vehicle road traffic collision and is unconscious. A bystander calls for an ambulance. **Paramedics** arrive on the scene and rapidly assess Paulina, determining that she is presenting with a right-sided midshaft femur fracture and bilateral tension pneumothoraces.

Paramedics provide critical pre-hospital interventions, such as oxygenation, bilateral thoracentesis, and application of a femoral traction splint. The paramedics transport Paulina to the nearest major trauma centre where they hand over Paulina's information and condition to the hospital's multidisciplinary team (MDT).

Doctors lead the trauma response, coordinating with **nurses** who offer urgent care and assist with procedures. **Surgeons** perform the necessary surgical interventions, such as a chest drain, while **anaesthetists** control pain during surgeries.

Radiographers conduct imaging studies to assess injuries through the use of CT scans. Once Paulina has been stabilised and started recovering, **physiotherapists** will aid in post-injury rehabilitation, helping Paulina regain mobility and strength.

Once discharged, **pharmacists** will ensure the proper management of medications and pain relief, and **occupational therapists** will help Paulina regain everyday skills and adapt to new limitations.

This collaborative MDT approach addresses the patient's short-, mid- and long-term needs, working together seamlessly to achieve the best patient outcomes possible.

6.2 Example B: Mental health

Arisu is experiencing a severe mental health crisis. He calls 999 for help, fearing he might harm himself.

Paramedics perform an assessment; they determine that Arisu needs immediate intervention and transfer him safely to the appropriate mental health hospital. They hand over care to the **emergency department team**.

A **mental health liaison nurse** assesses Arisu upon arrival, identifying signs of severe depression and anxiety. The nurse escalates Arisu's care to a psychiatrist.

The **psychiatrist** recommends admission to the psychiatric ward for further evaluation and treatment.

An **occupational therapist** and a **psychologist** work together to develop a comprehensive care plan for Arisu. The occupational therapist helps Arisu regain daily living skills and adapt to his current situation while the psychologist provides therapeutic interventions.

Arisu receives a **social worker** who addresses social determinants of health, such as housing and employment, ensuring that Arisu's social needs are met.

The social worker also facilitates Arisu's access to helpful **community resources**. Throughout Arisu's stay, the MDT collaborates to provide holistic care.

Family members are engaged in the care process, offering additional support while respecting Arisu's confidentiality and autonomy.

This collaborative MDT approach ensures that Arisu receives comprehensive care tailored to his unique needs, improving his overall mental health outcome. Arisu and his family are also key members of the team; they can advocate for his needs and ensure his wishes are heard. For more on working alongside service users, see *Section 18*.

6.3 Example C: Obstetric emergency

Susie is in labour. She calls 999, fearing she cannot get to the hospital in time. **Paramedics** perform an assessment; no abnormalities are identified at this stage, and they transfer Susie safely to the labour ward.

They hand over care to a **midwife**, who cares for Susie during her labour. Abnormalities are identified in the fetal heart rate, and care is escalated to an **obstetrician**. The obstetrician recommends an emergency caesarean birth, and Susie is transferred to the theatre, accompanied by the midwife.

An **anaesthetist** and **operating department practitioner** work together to provide anaesthesia and monitor Susie throughout the caesarean birth, which is performed by the obstetrician.

A **scrub midwife** and **healthcare support worker** support the medical team.

Paediatricians are paged to assess the baby at birth; the baby is well, and care is resumed by the midwife.

The midwife cares for Susie and baby in recovery before they are transferred to the **postnatal ward** for further monitoring.

The MDT ensures the safe delivery of Susie's baby by providing timely assessments, escalating care when complications arise, and coordinating emergency interventions. Their collaborative efforts support both mother and baby throughout labour, surgery and postnatal recovery, ensuring the best possible outcomes.

6.4 Example D: Disability and rehabilitation

Liam, a young boy, has experienced a traumatic brain injury following a fall.

Paramedics arrive promptly, assess his condition, and transport him to the nearest children's hospital, handing care to the **children's emergency department team**.

A **neurologist** evaluates Liam, determining the extent of his injury.

A **physiotherapist** and an **occupational therapist** collaborate to create a rehabilitation plan. The physiotherapist helps Liam regain mobility while the occupational therapist assists him in relearning daily activities.

A **speech and language therapist** works with Liam to address communication difficulties, providing therapy to improve his speech and swallowing functions.

A **psychologist** offers emotional support and therapeutic interventions to help Liam and his family cope with the psychological impact of the injury.

A **social worker** addresses social determinants of health, such as school reintegration and family support, ensuring Liam's social needs are met and facilitating access to community resources.

This MDT approach ensures Liam receives comprehensive, tailored care, enhancing his recovery and overall wellbeing.

Use the space below to make brief notes on the situations that you see involving an MDT approach in your practice:

Notes

7 Student roles within the MDT

7.1 Getting involved

Aim to be an '**active participant**'. To do this, students should aim to be more than just observers in MDT meetings, as contributing helps you to feel part of the team, creating a sense of belonging. This builds your self-esteem and self-worth, helping you feel motivated and enthusiastic about your role as a student professional.

You can **get involved** by asking questions and sharing insights with other professionals, to broaden their knowledge of the area you are working in and vice versa. This will help to bridge the gap between what you know and what you would like to know more about.

You can use this approach to help **create learning opportunities** with members of the MDT outside of your current placement area.

7.2 Expectations for students in the MDT

While engaging in MDTs, you are expected to demonstrate **professionalism**, active **participation** and a **willingness to learn**.

- Professionalism can be demonstrated by adhering to the dress code, being punctual and maintaining confidentiality.
- Participating in a meeting gives you the opportunity to showcase your effective communication active listening and questioning skills.
- Demonstrate your willingness to learn by researching in advance the professionals who are likely to be at the meeting, so you have an idea of their roles. *Section 2* can help you with this.

- Reflective writing about learning experiences helps to reinforce learning and provide evidence that this learning has happened, and allows you to revisit the experience. *Section 21* can help you with this.

Lastly, you should respect and value the contributions of all team members regardless of their profession, and they should respect yours too.

7.3 Benefits of involvement

Participating in an MDT meeting offers you numerous advantages that can enhance your learning and professional development.

- Practical learning: MDTs allow you to apply what you've learnt in the classroom to real-life situations. This hands-on experience helps bridge the gap between theory and practice, making learning more meaningful and relevant.
- Professional development: joining an MDT boosts confidence by showing the importance of each role. It helps gain a deeper understanding of your chosen discipline, which will help you to make relevant referrals in the future. For more on professional development, see *Section 20*.
- Interpersonal growth: working alongside professionals from various fields helps you to develop essential communication, teamwork and problem-solving skills. These experiences teach you how to collaborate effectively, adapt to different perspectives, and find solutions together.
- Networking: MDTs provide valuable opportunities to connect with professionals from various disciplines. Building these relationships can be helpful for mentorship, career advice, and even future job opportunities.

7.4 Involvement challenges (and solutions)

Despite the benefits, you may occasionally face challenges when working in an MDT, but they can be overcome.

Below you'll find some common challenges with suggested solutions alongside; there's also space to add some of your own.

Challenge	Solution
Feeling intimidated – the presence of experienced professionals can be overwhelming, causing students to feel unsure of their contributions	**Seek mentorship** – engaging with mentors can provide guidance, boost confidence, and clarify any uncertainties. For more on team integration, see *Section 9*
Knowledge gaps – you may find keeping up with technical terms or clinical discussions difficult at times, especially when less familiar with certain areas of expertise	**Ask questions** – actively seeking help or clarification fosters learning and helps bridge knowledge gaps
Miscommunication – finding the right words or expressing oneself assertively can be tough, particularly when communication styles differ across disciplines	**Reflect on experiences** – reflecting regularly allows you to identify areas of improvement. For more specifically on communication, see *Section 10*

By embracing these strategies, you can effectively navigate challenges, turn them into learning opportunities, and thrive within MDTs.

7.5 Practical tips

- Be **proactive** and **plan ahead**. Before going into a practice area, you can research about the common disciplines and team members you'll expect to see.
- **Research potential learning opportunities** that may be available in your placement area and wider MDTs to get the most out of your time there.
- Seek **feedback** which helps to improve your performance and promotes 'active learning' in the practice environment.
- Practice **active participation and learning** to develop critical thinking, problem-solving and decision-making skills.
- Keep a **reflective journal** or portfolio to document learning and growth – we learn from *reflecting* on experiences, not just the experiences themselves.

Add any other tips you note as you work in MDTs:

_____

_____

_____

_____

_____

_____

8 Building confidence

Building your confidence when working in an MDT is a gradual process that can be normalised through consistent practice and peer support.

Remember that you have been invited for a reason, and your unique perspective on things may differ from others' but is just as valuable.

Every team may have subtle or unsubtle differences, a different communication approach, and different professional jargon. However, adapting to the basic principles of MDT working will allow for more seamless collaboration over time.

8.1 Speaking up

Speaking up in an MDT can be daunting but is an effective way to raise your visibility in a team and build relationships with colleagues.

It is easy to overthink questions before asking them, which can mean the question is no longer relevant to the current discussions, so confidence is essential. But always remember to think first and consider whether your comment/question will add value or may best be discussed outside of the MDT.

Being confident in an MDT will take time, and everyone gets there in their own time, so don't be afraid if you feel it is a slow process or worry about making mistakes. It might help to know that everyone makes mistakes occasionally, but fostering a growth mindset ensures continuous development of mental wellbeing and skills as a student professional.

8.2 Reflecting on mistakes

Mistakes offer feedback that can be used to improve outcomes in subsequent MDT experiences.

Taking care of your wellbeing by getting sufficient sleep, maintaining a balanced diet, and practising mindfulness can help promote mental positivity and resilience within the ever-changing and challenging landscape of multidisciplinary working. One way this can be done is through reflections.

Reflection is an essential part of being a student and beneficial in supporting development when you go into practice. Many different reflective models can be used; it's worth spending time identifying one that would work best for you.

Reflective practice can help build strengths and identify areas for improvement, supporting your learning, growth and development personally and professionally.

Taking time to reflect on experiences provides an opportunity to develop self-awareness, learn from any mistakes, and become more resilient to the challenges faced in practice. This, in turn, can help you become a better advocate by encouraging you to ask questions and raise concerns, which can help build better communication between professionals.

8.3 Supporting patients to be confident

For the patient, your interaction with them could be a part of a more significant journey with many different professionals being involved.

Whilst your impact has the potential to be influential, it can be hard to explain and reassure patients what could be happening next for them if you are not aware of other team member roles.

When working in an MDT, it is essential to listen to what others are doing to help understand the bigger picture of the patient's journey with the team and also contribute to discussions.

8.4 Ways to build confidence

Seeking opportunities to shadow other professionals can support building confidence by reinforcing understanding of roles.

Shadowing others will help to enable you, as the learner, to get a sense of that profession's role and how something you may have noticed/referred to gets carried forward by another profession.

This can also highlight areas for improvement either in your practice or the culture as a whole. This is especially true regarding the importance of effective communication and how any breakdown can affect effective teamwork and, most importantly, patient outcomes and patient safety. For more on communication, see *Section 10*.

In high-stress environments, it may feel tough that you may not be the one to deliver the care a patient needs. However, knowing what another professional can do and being able to reassure your patients helps remind you all that you are working towards a shared goal.

Below you can find our top tips for building your confidence, with space for you to add your own and for you to note down how you've been able to complete the tips in the past.

Top tips

Our top tips	Example of when and how I've been able to do this
Introduce yourself to the team	
Speak to a colleague to gain understanding before a meeting	
Take time to speak to people	
Active listening	
Check your understanding	
Take notes	
Reflect on experiences	
Take care of your mental and physical wellbeing	
Remember, you have been invited for a reason	

Collaborative working within the MDT

- **9.** Integrating into teams 36
- **10.** Communication strategies to support integration 39
- **11.** Civility 44
- **12.** Inclusivity and teamwork within care 48
- **13.** Managing differing priorities and potential conflict 52
- **14.** Use of language 57
- **15.** MDT working: Good practice advice 59

9 Integrating into teams

Why is team integration so important?

- It is important to feel part of a team when collaborative working is such a core part of improving patient care and satisfaction outcomes.
- There is a wide body of literature that supports interprofessional collaboration (IPC) between professionals, which has been linked to an increase in patient quality of life (more specifically, psychiatric and physical functioning ability) and improved management of their own health care, as well as improved staff/patient relationships and overall treatment success.
- Having that sense of belonging within a team/department means you are more likely to work reliably and increase in confidence and, in turn, capability.
- Students who felt included and trusted are more likely to develop their professional competency and identity of what each person brings to the team.
- Fundamentally, team integration preserves your human dignity as a student professional with feelings, opinions and potentially untapped potential instead of being labelled as 'the student'.

9.1 What are the benefits to staff and patient care?

Benefits to patient care

By integrating into teams, comprehensive and holistic care is ensured, drawing together different professionals' knowledge to address multiple aspects of patients' health, meaning no area of patient care is overlooked.

This collaboration encourages more accurate diagnoses and timely treatments whilst monitoring and adjustment of care plans is more effective, so all the needs of patients are continuously met.

Efficiency in teamwork means interventions can be provided quickly in emergency situations, reducing the risk of delayed care negatively impacting prognosis. This builds up rapport and fosters trust and satisfaction, as better coordination minimises risk of errors, duplication and miscommunication.

Add any other benefits you have noticed as you work in MDTs:

_____

_____

_____

_____

Benefits to staff (including you!)

- Teamwork promotes more open communication, which initiates a more supportive work environment, where the joint resolution of issues reduces individual stress.
- Working within a diverse team exposes staff to different levels of skills, expertise and experiences, fostering professional development.
- Learning from one another leads to better competence and allows for better thought-out solutions through a shared decision-making process.
- Not only does this promote continuous learning but it also reduces burnout. Being part of a team can reduce emotional strain, common amongst those working in health and social care, and provide the support of a team to lean on.

9.2 Potential difficulties of integrating when you are 'the student'

Integrating into MDTs as a student can be challenging for many reasons, such as perceived hierarchies or a lack of confidence.

Students sometimes experience imposter syndrome and feel overlooked and are hesitant to contribute, which can limit participation.

Practical ways to overcome difficulties

- Build confidence through active participation. For more information about building confidence, see *Section 8*.
- Prepare for team discussions in advance. Read through patient notes so you are prepared; researching anything you are unsure of will enable you to contribute more confidently. Using tools such as SBAR can help with this. For more about communication tools, see *Section 10*.
- Ask your supervisor or another member of the team for guidance and support. Doing this can offer a safe space to ask questions and develop your professional skills.

Another challenge students encounter while integrating into MDTs is the difficulty in establishing their role and demonstrating their value within the team.

As a student, you might feel unsure about how your contributions help with patient care; this can lead to missed opportunities to participate. To overcome this, you can focus on proactively clarifying your role and responsibilities with your supervisor at the beginning of each placement.

Ask the team you're working with about specific responsibilities they expect you to undertake, which can also demonstrate your willingness to learn and develop. For more about student expectations within MDT working see *Section 7*, and for more about communication techniques that can help you integrate within the team see *Section 10*.

Communication strategies to support integration

Effective communication is critical for students integrating into MDTs.

It ensures accurate information exchange, supports collaborative decision-making, and safeguards patient safety.

For students, engaging in effective communication allows you to actively participate, bridge knowledge gaps, and establish your professional identity within a team.

Using strategies such as SBAR for specific tasks – such as a handover – alongside active listening techniques can help you navigate the complexities of MDTs and deliver patient-centred care.

10.1 SBAR

SBAR (Situation, Background, Assessment, Recommendation) (NHS Improvement, 2017) is a key NHS communication tool that helps students deliver concise, logical handovers and escalate concerns effectively.

In many settings, SBAR can enhance communication and teamwork.

Digital tools such as **electronic health records** (EHRs) and secure messaging systems streamline information sharing and ensure continuity of care. These platforms enhance team coordination and address privacy concerns critical for trust.

Situation	Briefly describe the current situation or issue (e.g. *"The patient is experiencing shortness of breath"*)
Background	Provide relevant background information (e.g. *"The patient has a history of COPD and was recently admitted for pneumonia"*)
Assessment	Share your assessment or interpretation of the situation (e.g. *"Oxygen saturation is dropping, and the patient appears fatigued"*)
Recommendation	Offer your suggestion for action or request further evaluation (e.g. *"I recommend increasing oxygen flow or considering a chest X-ray"*)

10.2 Demonstrating active listening and assertiveness

Active listening helps you to navigate MDTs by understanding others' perspectives, ensuring clarity, and demonstrating empathy.

Techniques such as maintaining eye contact, paraphrasing, and asking clarifying questions build trust and show respect within the team.

Below are two techniques to help demonstrate your active listening skills that you may wish to try.

SOLER technique

SOLER (Egan, 2014) is a communication method for active listening and non-verbal engagement.

Sit squarely	Position yourself facing the person, showing attentiveness
Open posture	Keep your body open, avoiding crossed arms to show receptivity
Lean forward	Demonstrate interest by leaning slightly towards the speaker
Eye contact	Maintain appropriate eye contact to convey focus and empathy
Relax	Stay calm and relaxed, as tension can hinder effective communication

SURETY technique

SURETY (Stickley, 2011) is a method for establishing trust and credibility in communication.

Sit at an angle	Position yourself at an angle to the person, creating a non-confrontational stance
Uncross arms and legs	Avoid closed-off body language to make the other person feel comfortable
Relax	Maintain a relaxed posture to reduce stress and foster openness
Eye contact	Maintain steady, respectful eye contact, showing engagement
Touch	If and when appropriate, a gentle touch can demonstrate empathy and connection
Your full attention	Give the person your full attention, without distractions

Assertiveness allows you to share ideas confidently and contribute to decision-making without aggression. Using respectful language, a steady voice, and "I" statements helps to express concerns and insights, ensuring care remains person-centred.

These skills can empower you to engage meaningfully in MDTs, enhancing collaboration and reinforcing your professional identity. For more on professional identity, see *Section 16*.

10.3 Understanding hierarchies and overcoming communication barriers to build relationships

Health and social care hierarchies rank individuals by authority, status or expertise, which can feel intimidating for students.

Every role, *including yours*, brings value to MDTs, and contributions are important for team success.

You may find it challenging to voice your thoughts, but tools such as SBAR, SOLER and SURETY provide structure to articulate concerns confidently and showcase your active listening.

Informal conversations with team members also foster rapport, break down barriers, and help you feel more integrated into the team. These experiences enable students to navigate hierarchies and grow professionally within MDTs.

Building relationships within the MDT

Building strong relationships within MDTs helps you establish trust and foster collaboration. Active participation in discussions, showing respect, and demonstrating a willingness to learn are key strategies.

Simple actions – such as being prepared, listening attentively and acknowledging others' contributions – convey professionalism and mutual respect.

You can also create connections through informal interactions, such as shadowing colleagues or asking questions during quiet moments.

Seeking feedback and maintaining a proactive attitude shows your value as a contributor, helping you integrate confidently into the team and build networks that enhance collaboration and patient care.

Key takeaways

Effective communication is essential for you to integrate into MDTs, enabling you to contribute meaningfully, build professional relationships and ensure patient safety.

By adopting structured tools such as SBAR, practising active listening through SOLER/SURETY and being appropriately assertive, you can navigate the complexities of MDTs with confidence.

Notes

Egan, G. (2014) *The Skilled Helper: a problem-management and opportunity-development approach to helping*, 10th edition. Cengage Learning.

NHS Improvement (2017) *SBAR: situation, background, assessment, recommendation – implementation and training guide*. Available at: www.england.nhs.uk/improvement-hub/wp-content/uploads/sites/44/2017/11/SBAR-Implementation-and-Training-Guide.pdf

Stickley, T. (2011) From SOLER to SURETY for therapeutic communication. *Nursing Times*, 107(48): 18–19.

11. Civility

For health and social care practitioners, **civility refers to our attitudes to and respect for one another**, the way in which we treat each other at work.

Civility begins with actively listening to and valuing the input of all our colleagues. Recognising and respecting the unique experience of each team member can enhance our decision-making and strengthen the quality of the care we provide.

Civility means maintaining professional behaviour even when faced with challenging situations; for example, taking part in high-pressure clinical discussions. In such situations civility can be achieved by using clear, respectful language and by offering constructive contributions.

Final year Midwifery students in one of the author's universities were asked what civility means to them, and came up with the following word cloud:

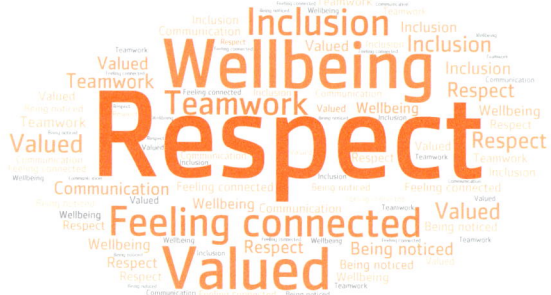

Civility is essential in fostering effective teamwork, promoting collaboration and in improving patient care and outcomes. Thus, civility has been placed at the heart of future planning for the NHS.

Current NHS policies emphasise kindness, compassion and respect in practice, to create a supportive and inclusive culture for staff and patients. The current 10 Year Health Plan highlights a requirement for instances of incivility to reduce, in order for the NHS to succeed as a service and employer.

Incorporating civility into your daily practice aligns with the NHS Constitution's core values of respect and dignity. Healthcare professionals modelling civility set the tone for their teams, creating a positive working culture that supports patient and colleague safety, along with the open exchange of ideas – key ingredients for implementing excellent, patient-centred care.

11.1 The Civility Saves Lives campaign

This campaign highlights the profound impact of civility upon error reduction and improvement of patient safety; it emphasises that small actions – such as thanking colleagues or offering support during stressful experiences – bolster the foundations of a positive work environment.

Incivility, which can take the form of bullying, harassment, rudeness or unkindness, can unfortunately become common in high-pressure environments. Just because incivility can become commonplace does not make it acceptable.

Civility Saves Lives reports that people who witness incivility can experience a 20% decrease in performance at work, whilst 25% of recipients of incivility take this out on service users. Students experiencing incivility on placement also report lower compliance with safety precautions such as following hand hygiene protocols.

For more about the campaign, please visit www.civilitysaveslives.com.

11.2 Acting on civility

Explore the resources in this section to learn more about civility in health care and how you can incorporate civility into your practice as a health and social care professional working within MDTs.

 Activity

> **Read:** the code of practice for your professional body – does it make reference to civility or its concepts?
>
> **Watch:** Chris Turner's TEDxExeter Talk, *When rudeness in teams turns deadly*, at bit.ly/3EHz2e7
>
> **Do:** explore the Royal College of Obstetricians and Gynaecologists (RCOG) Workplace Behaviour Toolkit, at bit.ly/4d5Vo5z
>
> This toolkit will help you to understand more about workplace behaviours and the impact of incivility on the people in our care. It includes tools to help develop your confidence in speaking up when necessary and in addressing poor workplace behaviours.
>
> We recommend starting with Module 7: *I want to learn more about workplace behaviour*.

Use the space below to record your thoughts:

Notes

12 Inclusivity and teamwork within care

Inclusivity means ensuring that all team members, regardless of their background or expertise, are allowed to contribute meaningfully, promoting holistic approaches to patient care.

Inclusivity is a vital element within teamwork and health care. All healthcare professionals should value the diverse perspectives, skills and experiences of those involved in an MDT.

12.1 Key principles of inclusivity and teamwork

- **Communication:** clear, open communication is essential. Team members must share information openly and listen to each other to ensure that everyone understands what is being discussed. Barriers to communication, such as using medical jargon or not making reasonable adjustments for those with communication difficulties, can limit this inclusivity and can hinder the professional relationship between you and the team around you, and most importantly the person the MDT is about. For more on communication, see *Section 10*.
- **Respect:** every member brings unique expertise. Recognising and respecting each role, whether it's a doctor, nurse, social worker or unpaid carer, can help to build trust within the team.
- **Shared goals:** all team members should be focused on the same patient-centred goals. Whether it's improving patient outcomes or reducing hospital readmissions, having common objectives helps guide teamwork.

- **Collaboration:** teams must work together, using each member's strengths. Collaboration means coordinating care and offering support when needed.

12.2 Benefits of inclusivity and teamwork

When health and social care professionals work together seamlessly, patient care improves.

Team members can catch potential issues early, offer more holistic care, and ensure that all aspects of a patient's health are considered.

Not feeling part of a team can impact on communication, which can then impact on the effectiveness of the team and patient care. Health and social care workers who, conversely, have felt part of a team had a sense of belonging which contributed towards their personal growth.

Health and social care are focused on empowering patients to help support them in their recovery and improve their wellbeing, and by promoting an inclusive environment with patients, you can improve communication, allowing you to work more effectively with patients and achieve their needs and the needs of the team more quickly.

12.3 Challenges facing inclusivity and teamwork

There are many challenges that prevent a team from working effectively, therefore not providing effective care.

- **Power dynamics:** in health care, for example, there is sometimes an assumption that doctors often hold more authority than nurses or other team members. This can make it difficult for some professionals to speak up. To overcome this, teams need to encourage and develop cultures where contribution from all roles is equally valued.

- **Time constraints:** professionals often work to tight timeframes, making it hard to find time to involve all professionals in their decision-making. Regular meetings or use of digital tools for communication can help overcome this barrier.
- **Bias and prejudice:** personal biases, whether related to gender, race or professional status, can affect how team members work together. Addressing bias and prejudices through training can help eliminate this within a team, facilitating an effective bias-free working environment.

12.4 Building an inclusive team environment

This involves creating a culture where every individual feels respected and valued.

- **Encouraging participation:** every team member should feel encouraged to contribute ideas and solutions.
- **Defined roles and responsibilities:** clear role definition helps prevent confusion and ensures that all team members understand their responsibilities in patient care.
- **Regular team meetings:** regular check-ins or meetings allow the team to align patient care plans, discuss challenges facing care, and share recent developments.
- **Removing barriers:** removing barriers and bias helps create a truly inclusive environment for collaboration.
- **Providing equal opportunities:** this allows for participation and development, which makes individuals feel valued and lays the foundation for further participation in the future.

Add any other strategies you have noticed as you work in MDTs:

_____

_____

_____

_____

✎ Notes

13 Managing differing priorities and potential conflict

Professionals across various disciplines are frequently required to balance competing priorities.

These priorities range from urgent and non-urgent needs to acute and chronic conditions, requiring coordinated multidisciplinary collaboration to ensure holistic, patient-centred care.

Understanding how different professionals contribute to managing these diverse priorities is key to effective health and social care delivery.

13.1 Balancing urgent and non-urgent needs

Urgent care involves immediate interventions to prevent deterioration or life-threatening outcomes. Examples include heart attacks, strokes, acute psychotic episodes, or safeguarding concerns for a person with a learning disability.

In contrast, non-urgent care includes routine check-ups, long-term condition management, and preventive measures such as vaccinations and health education.

Understanding urgent and non-urgent needs will help with prioritising care. There is space below for you to add additional examples you've seen.

- **Examples of urgent care professionals:** paramedics, emergency physicians and acute medical teams prioritise urgent cases, ensuring timely life-saving interventions.

Mental health crisis teams perform a similar role for patients experiencing psychiatric emergencies.

_____

_____

- **Examples of non-urgent care professionals:** general practitioners (GPs), district nurses and social workers address non-urgent but essential care needs, such as medication management, therapy referrals and social support.

_____

_____

Managing acute vs. chronic conditions

Acute conditions are sudden and severe, while chronic conditions persist over time and require ongoing management. Navigating both types requires seamless coordination among professionals to prevent acute exacerbations of chronic illnesses and ensure continuity of care.

- **Examples of acute conditions:** myocardial infarction, pneumonia, acute psychosis and epilepsy seizures demand rapid response and intensive treatment from emergency services, hospital specialists and psychiatric crisis teams.

_____

_____

- **Examples of chronic conditions:** diabetes, schizophrenia, dementia and autism spectrum disorders necessitate long-term engagement from multidisciplinary teams, including GPs, mental health professionals, learning disability nurses and social care workers.

___

___

13.2 Managing differing priorities in an MDT

In MDTs, professionals bring distinct expertise, perspectives and priorities. These differences are valuable but can also create challenges when deciding the best course of action for a patient. Effective communication, shared decision-making and professional respect help manage these differing priorities.

Prioritisation strategies in MDTs

1. Triage and risk assessment
   - Using structured tools, such as the National Early Warning Score (NEWS2) for physical health or the Threshold Assessment Grid (TAG) for mental health, can help identify the most pressing needs.
   - Regular team meetings and handovers ensure that all professionals understand current priorities.
2. Person-centred care
   - The patient's goals and preferences should guide decision-making, ensuring care aligns with their needs and values.
   - Engaging family members or carers (where appropriate) can help in understanding long-term priorities beyond immediate medical concerns.

3. Flexible working approaches
   - Professionals must be adaptable, recognising when immediate medical intervention is needed versus when long-term social support should take priority.
   - Collaboration is key – district nurses, for instance, may adjust their schedules to accommodate urgent mental health reviews.

13.3 Potential conflict in MDTs

Disagreements may arise when professionals have differing views on what should take priority. Common sources of conflict include:

- Resource allocation: limited staffing or funding may mean that not all interventions can be provided immediately.
- Professional perspectives: a social worker may advocate for long-term housing solutions, while a doctor may prioritise urgent medical treatment.
- Ethical dilemmas: differences in opinion regarding capacity, consent or safeguarding concerns can create tension.

Conflict resolution in MDTs

1. Active listening and open communication
   - Encourage each professional to articulate their concerns and rationale without interruption.
   - Use structured discussions, such as SBAR (see *Section 10.1*), to present differing viewpoints clearly.
2. Negotiation and compromise
   - Aim for solutions that balance urgent needs with long-term care planning.
   - Where possible, create shared action plans that accommodate multiple priorities.

3. Escalation pathways
   - When consensus cannot be reached, referring to senior colleagues, clinical leads or ethics committees can provide additional guidance.
   - Clear escalation policies ensure timely decision-making without unnecessary delays in care.
4. Interprofessional education and reflection
   - Learning about each other's roles and responsibilities helps prevent misunderstandings.
   - Reflective practice, such as debriefing after challenging MDT meetings, strengthens future collaboration.

Use the space below to note any other conflict resolution approaches you have seen:

_____

_____

_____

_____

_____

_____

_____

_____

Use of language

Effective communication within an MDT is essential, but challenges can arise when different disciplines use the same terms with varying meanings. Clarity in language ensures that professionals understand each other and work towards shared goals.

Language is a dynamic and essential concept in health care, shaping the understanding of clinical contexts and informing practice across multiple professional fields.

A key challenge arises in the terminology used across these fields, as specific terms can carry vastly different meanings depending on the professional context.

14.1 Common language barriers in MDTs

Same terms, different meanings
- 'Observation' in **adult nursing** often refers to monitoring a patient's vital signs, while in **mental health nursing**, it may mean direct supervision of a high-risk patient.
- 'Review' in **social care** may mean a routine assessment of care needs, but for a **doctor**, it could mean an urgent reassessment of treatment.

Use of jargon and acronyms
- Different professions have their own terminology, which can be confusing for colleagues from other disciplines.

Professional bias in communication
- Language can sometimes reflect unconscious bias, such as using medicalised terms when discussing social issues or vice versa.
- Using neutral, patient-centred language ensures inclusivity and collaboration.

14.2 Strategies for clear communication and language

Clarification and standardisation
- Teams should agree on shared definitions of key terms during MDT meetings, to avoid misinterpretation.
- Asking for clarification when unfamiliar terms arise fosters a culture of learning and respect.

Using structured communication tools
- SBAR, for example, helps standardise communication and reduce misunderstandings (see *Section 10.1*).
- Plain language summaries should be used when discussing care plans with colleagues from different disciplines.

Active listening and feedback
- Encouraging professionals to reflect on what has been said ensures mutual understanding.
- MDTs should promote a culture where asking questions is welcomed and encouraged.

Training and interprofessional learning
- Joint training sessions on communication improve understanding of different professional languages.
- Role-playing common scenarios helps MDT members develop confidence in addressing language barriers.

By recognising differences in terminology, reducing jargon, and promoting clear communication, professionals can collaborate more effectively and ensure that all team members are aligned in their approach to patient-centred care.

15 MDT working: Good practice advice

Continuous improvement

- Continuous improvement, time management and efficiency are vital for MDT effectiveness. Good practice involves skills such as leadership, processes such as governance, and critical values such as respect and patient centrality.
- Continuous improvement focuses on ongoing service or individual practice enhancements, targeting both processes and cultures. Good practice in nursing and MDT work, for example, can reduce patient complaints, lower hospital mortality rates, and increase staff satisfaction and health.
- Using SMART (Specific, Measurable, Achievable, Relevant and Time-bound) goals helps identify specific targets and ways to achieve them. Support for improving NHS services includes initiatives such as 'Always Events', which incorporate patients' views, and the NHS Leadership Qualities Framework (see figure), outlining desirable traits for continuous improvement.
- Managing MDT culture is crucial, as incivility can harm patients and team effectiveness. Good communication, awareness of actions, and a positive perspective are essential.
- The 6Cs in health care – a set of values for all health and social care staff, comprising Compassion, Communication, Care, Courage, Commitment and Competence – should guide the team's efforts.

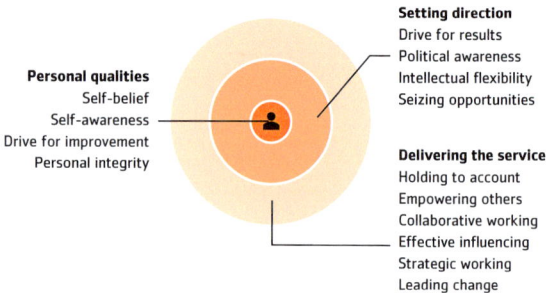

Figure based on the Leadership Qualities Framework (NHS Leadership Academy, 2011).

Adaptability and flexibility

- Adaptability and flexibility are crucial for effective MDTs in health and social care.
- Each team member, including the patient, may have different commitments, so accommodating their concerns and needs is essential.
- Online meetings can save time and offer flexibility, but it's important to be mindful of digital literacy, digital poverty and confidentiality. Ensuring that all participants are in a secure environment to discuss confidential information is vital.
- Consistent scheduling, such as setting meetings at the same day and time each week, can help. Setting an agenda for MDT meetings ensures priorities are addressed and space is provided for the patient to express concerns.

NHS Leadership Academy (2011) *The Leadership Framework*. Available at: bit.ly/3YzpZTd

Use the space below to note examples you have observed or where you have demonstrated adaptability and flexibility:

_____

_____

_____

Notes

Enhancing the MDT experience

16. Professional identity 64

17. Collaboration with stakeholders 67

18. Co-production with patients/service users. 70

19. Patient safety 73

20. Professional development opportunities. 78

21. Scenarios for guided reflection and action planning. 81

22. Further understanding: ethics and integrity in MDT working 86

23. The importance of self-care for health and social care professionals working within the MDT. 90

16   Professional identity

Professional identity is the **self-concept based on attributes, beliefs, values, motives and experiences in one's profession**. In health and social care, a strong professional identity provides clarity in roles, ensuring effective collaboration within MDTs.

Foundations of professional identity

Professional identity develops through education, training and experience, shaping how individuals perceive their role and interact with others.

For MDTs, understanding how professional identity shapes team dynamics is crucial. Traditionally, those in certain professions, such as doctors, have been viewed as team leaders, but effective MDTs embrace shared leadership. Professionals must align their individual expertise with collective team goals to enhance patient care.

 Activity

> Briefly reflect on an experience where your professional identity was challenged or reinforced. How did it shape your understanding of your role?
>
> _____
>
> _____
>
> _____
>
> _____
>
> _____

16.1 The role of professional identity in MDT working

A well-defined professional identity helps prevent role confusion and ensures that team members understand their responsibilities.

- Role awareness and clarification: clear professional boundaries enhance collaboration (e.g. setting expectations at the start of a working situation).
- Mutual respect: encouraging an environment where all team members' skills and expertise are valued enhances collaboration and patient outcomes.
- Risks of stereotyping: making assumptions about roles can undermine team cohesion. For example, as a student, you may feel undervalued in certain MDT discussions.

16.2 Strengthening professional identity in MDTs

Developing a strong professional identity involves self-awareness and continuous learning.

Consider these suggested tasks to strengthen your own professional identity:

- Reflective practice tools: using reflective models, journalling or peer discussions help professionals critically assess their evolving identity. For more on reflection, see *Section 21*.
- Learning from role models: observing experienced professionals in MDT situations can help develop resilience and confidence in one's role.
- Opportunities for growth: multiprofessional placements, insight days and conferences broaden perspectives and reinforce identity.

- Mentorship: a strong mentor can help navigate professional challenges and encourage career development.

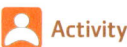
Activity

> Identify a mentor or professional who exemplifies strong professional identity. What key traits do they display?
>
> _____
>
> _____
>
> _____
>
> _____
>
> _____

Building a collaborative identity

Professional identity does not exist in isolation; it must integrate with the wider MDT to ensure patient-centred care.

- Blending individual and team identity: recognising the value of personal expertise while working towards collective goals
- Encouraging open communication: respecting diverse perspectives within MDTs fosters an inclusive working environment
- Empowering all team members: valuing contributions from all disciplines, regardless of seniority
- Patient-centred care: understanding how professional identity contributes to holistic care enhances outcomes.

Collaboration with stakeholders

Wider stakeholders in health and social care include individuals, groups or organisations that contribute to or are affected by health and social care delivery, policy and outcomes.

They extend beyond the core MDT and include patients and families, community and voluntary organisations, primary care networks, social care providers, policymakers and commissioners, education and training institutions, private sector and technology providers, public health bodies, and regulatory and legal stakeholders.

Each plays a vital role in ensuring coordinated care, addressing health and social needs, promoting safety, fostering innovation, and aligning care with policies and standards.

17.1 Key principles of collaboration with stakeholders

To be able to collaborate with stakeholders in the MDT and provide person-centred, high-quality care, it's important to understand some of the basics of collaboration and partnership.

Firstly, **mutual respect** is an essential aspect of collaboration. All involved should value the opinions and expertise of each other; this can be achieved through active listening and regular engagement with stakeholders.

Open communication can help to ensure that information flows clearly and effectively between all stakeholders; this promotes transparency and a mutual understanding of each other's roles.

Having a **shared goal** ensures that all stakeholders are working towards the same outcome, which helps to reduce conflicting priorities and promotes more effective collaboration. This also enhances communication, since the shared goal is the main topic of discussions, resulting in clearer communication.

Honesty and trust will allow all involved to build stronger working relationships, and allow stakeholders to rely on each other's expertise and judgement. This helps to reduce the risk of power imbalances, as each person will be able to see each other's contributions as important to achieving success.

Finally, **accountability** ensures that each stakeholder accepts responsibility for their role and engagement. Accountability is especially crucial as it guarantees that all actions and care are patient-centred and that any errors made are acknowledged, addressed and reflected on, allowing for continuous development.

Challenges and strategies

Collaboration with stakeholders can sometimes be difficult, especially as a student, because of communication barriers, power imbalances or conflicting goals.

- Communication barriers can become a challenge when, for example, different people use different terminologies or have a different understanding to you.
- The most important thing to remember is that clear communication is essential; try to encourage open dialogue.

It can also be useful to establish common goals from the beginning and continue revisiting these. This way you are all working towards the same outcome and all team members are united through this.

Additionally, colleague support and role clarity can help to further reduce power imbalances.

- Colleagues can support by providing guidance on any hierarchical structures, and having role clarity means you know exactly what is expected of you and can work towards this specific goal.

Top tips for collaboration

- The important thing to remember is that you, as a health and social care student, provide an important perspective, and your involvement has a lot of value.
- Strive to develop clear communication channels, establishing shared goals with stakeholders. See *Chapter 10* for more details.

Add your own tips as a reminder to yourself:

_____

_____

_____

_____

_____

18. Co-production with patients / service users

Co-production in health and social care refers to the approach professionals take to include patients, caregivers or other support networks and stakeholders to work together as equals in order to design, deliver and improve services.

There is also high value placed by the Care Quality Commission (CQC) and other organisations on the importance of contributions from people with lived experiences or 'Experts by Experience', which can be utilised to create positive change.

18.1 Core principles of co-production

Accessibility: considers the transparency or confidentiality of information and information sharing within an MDT or beyond.

- **In action:** highlights the importance of equity, so that approaches used or materials produced are widely usable and inclusive.

Diversity: allowing as many experiences as possible to be included with the appropriate understanding of consent or other ethical considerations to include populations such as those with learning disabilities.

- **In action:** reduces the risk of excluding individuals and lessens this within an MDT.

Reciprocity: respect is a key component because individuals' experiences or knowledge are worthy and have value.

- **In action:** this also focuses on how those with lived experience are recompensed for sharing their experiences, providing education or feedback.

Equality: creating partnerships whereby service users, stakeholders and healthcare professionals are all equal and work collaboratively without power imbalances.

- **In action:** decisions are shared and made jointly, and consider the perspectives of all those involved.

Challenges of co-production in MDTs

While co-production offers many benefits, it also presents challenges. A negative culture within an MDT, lack of trust in professionals, and the highly context-dependent nature of co-production can hinder its success. Additionally, compared to traditional approaches, it often requires more time and resources to implement effectively.

Examples in practice

As you read the examples, make notes on the process and potential impact of co-production and consider if it could be applied to MDT working in your placement area.

> **Example 1: Always events and virtual wards**
>
> As part of ongoing NHS initiatives, co-production has been used to create 'Always events' – specific aspects of care that all patients experience consistently. Similarly, the NHS has applied co-production principles in response to the Covid-19 pandemic, such as establishing virtual wards and using digital platforms for clinical appointments. These innovations were captured through the Beneficial Changes Network to influence future healthcare practices. This approach emphasises making co-production a standard practice, reducing inequalities, and fostering a culture of positive change and leadership.

Your notes:

___

___

___

___

Example 2: Communication and collaboration

Co-production principles help improve communication, empower individuals, and build strong relationships within an MDT, shifting the focus towards 'partnerships, not projects'. Clear communication involves three key stages: first, making individuals aware of their options; secondly, providing information on available choices; and thirdly, listening to preferences and supporting collaborative decision-making.

By involving service users in service design, co-production ensures that care remains patient-centred. Sharing power, trust and responsibility fosters engagement, making individuals more likely to collaborate in the future. This approach also helps break down barriers to accessing and shaping healthcare services.

Your notes:

___

___

___

___

Patient safety

Patient safety is a core principle of effective healthcare, requiring vigilance, teamwork and a commitment to excellence from all members of the MDT. It focuses on preventing errors and ensuring high-quality, safe care for every patient. In the UK, initiatives emphasise the shared responsibility of MDTs in maintaining and improving patient safety.

Understanding patient safety

Patient safety involves identifying, analysing and mitigating risks that may harm patients. Common safety challenges include the following:

- Medication errors: incorrect dosing, administering the wrong drug, or missed doses
- Communication breakdowns: misunderstandings between team members or incomplete handovers
- Infections: healthcare-associated infections, such as MRSA, due to inadequate hygiene practices
- Diagnostic delays or errors: misdiagnosis or delayed interventions impacting patient outcomes
- Falls and injuries: incidents within healthcare settings due to environmental hazards or inadequate supervision.

Note

Patient harm potentially reduces global economic growth by 0.7% per year.

These risks highlight the importance of a cohesive MDT approach to patient safety, ensuring that every team member contributes their expertise to prevent harm.

19.1 The role of the MDT in patient safety

MDTs bring together professionals with diverse skills and perspectives, fostering holistic care for patients. However, collaboration also introduces complexities that can impact safety.

Key roles within the MDT include the following:

- Nurses: often the first point of contact, nurses monitor patients' conditions and implement safety protocols.
- Doctors: diagnose and develop treatment plans, ensuring decisions are evidence-based and patient-centred.
- Pharmacists: oversee medication management, reducing the risk of errors and interactions.
- Allied Health Professionals (AHPs): provide specialised care (e.g. physiotherapy, occupational therapy) that enhances recovery and prevents complications.
- Support staff: ensure the clinical environment is safe, clean and well-equipped.

For MDTs to optimise patient safety, members must maintain open communication, mutual respect, and a shared understanding of safety priorities.

 Activity

> What additional MDT roles that impact patient safety have you seen?
>
> _____
> _____
> _____
> _____

Challenges in maintaining patient safety

Despite its importance, ensuring patient safety can be a challenge. Challenges include the following:

- Human factors: fatigue, stress and cognitive overload can impair decision-making and attention to detail.
- Systemic issues: insufficient staffing, outdated equipment or unclear protocols can compromise care.
- Cultural barriers: hierarchical dynamics or fear of speaking up may prevent the reporting of safety concerns.
- Complex cases: patients with multiple comorbidities require intricate care plans, increasing the potential for errors.

Recognising these challenges enables MDTs to proactively address vulnerabilities, enhancing safety outcomes.

19.2 Strategies for enhancing patient safety

- Promoting a safety culture:
  - Encourage open reporting of incidents and near-misses without fear of blame.
  - Regularly review and learn from adverse events to prevent recurrence.
  - Empower all team members to speak up about safety concerns.
- Effective communication:
  - Utilise standardised tools such as SBAR (see *Section 10.1*) for structured communication.
  - Implement clear handover procedures during shift changes and transitions of care.
- Training and education:
  - Provide ongoing training on patient safety principles, including infection control, medication safety and human factors.
  - Conduct simulation-based learning to practise managing high-risk scenarios.

- Risk assessment and management:
  - Perform regular risk assessments to identify potential hazards.
  - Develop and implement action plans to address identified risks.
- Use of technology:
  - Use electronic health records (EHRs) to improve information-sharing and reduce documentation errors.
  - Implement clinical decision support systems (CDSS) to guide evidence-based care.
- Interdisciplinary collaboration:
  - Foster teamwork through regular MDT meetings and case reviews.
  - Ensure that all team members understand their roles and responsibilities in maintaining safety.

Activity

What other strategies have you seen?

_____

_____

_____

Case study: learning from adverse events

Juan, a 72-year-old patient with diabetes and hypertension, was admitted for surgery. Postoperatively, Juan experienced hypoglycaemia due to an uncoordinated handover between the surgical and medical teams. Insulin administration continued without accounting for reduced oral intake. A root cause analysis revealed gaps in communication during the handover process.

Before reading the text below, consider what lessons could be learned from this example:

_____

_____

_____

Lessons learned:
- A standardised handover protocol was introduced, ensuring critical information about Juan's medications and dietary needs was communicated clearly.
- Staff received training on recognising and managing hypoglycaemia.
- Regular audits were conducted to monitor adherence to the new protocol.

This case highlights the importance of learning from adverse events and implementing system-wide improvements to enhance patient safety.

Patient safety is a shared responsibility that lies at the heart of MDT practice. By fostering a culture of openness, continuous learning and collaboration, MDTs can minimise risks and provide safer care for patients.

Through collective commitment to safety, health and social care professionals not only protect their patients but also enhance trust and confidence in the health and social care system.

20 Professional development opportunities

Continuing professional development (CPD) is a cornerstone to the success of MDTs in health care.

A commitment to continuous learning underpins the effective function of MDTs, enabling team members to collaborate seamlessly in order to deliver comprehensive, patient-centred care.

By developing a deeper understanding of your role and that of others within the team, professional development can help reduce role overlaps and miscommunication, ultimately streamlining the workflow of every team member and improving overall efficiency.

- On an **individual level,** professional development builds both confidence and competence. Team members can equip themselves with the tools to stay apace with the ever-evolving demands of their various disciplines.
- On a **team level,** it strengthens the collective problem-solving capabilities and reinforces the fundamentals of shared decision-making. This not only enhances a team's cohesion, but leads to measurable improvements in patient outcomes, including markedly fewer errors and more timely interventions.

The NHS Signpost for CPD also underlines the importance of fostering interprofessional learning, particularly as a strategy for addressing healthcare challenges in the near future. Taking advantage of today's developing technologies, initiatives can focus on collaborative training and professional growth, empowering teams to adapt to the rapidly evolving landscape of health care; ensuring that they remain at the forefront of care excellence and innovation.

By investing in professional development, members of the MDT can continue to provide the high-quality care that is essential for meeting complex patient needs.

20.1 Types of professional development opportunities for MDT members

The majority of members of the MDT – whether they are medics, nurses, midwives or other allied health professionals – will be regulated by a professional body which provides both formal and informal opportunities for CPD.

Some MDT members may be required to complete a certain amount of CPD by their professional body, as is the case with the Nursing and Midwifery Council (NMC), which requires its members to complete 35 hours of CPD every 3 years in order to be revalidated and remain on their nursing register. Ways of meeting this requirement vary, from accredited courses to online discussion groups and consultations.

Other bodies may not have such requirements but still offer opportunities for their members to undertake CPD, such as the Royal College of Speech and Language Therapists, which partners with Clinical Excellence Networks (CENs) to provide clinicians with opportunities to share evidence-based practice or participate in training as part of their professional development in a specialist area of practice.

Interprofessional education (IPE), where different members of the MDT learn and train together, is also invaluable for the effective functioning of the MDT, helping to build relationships across professions and enabling clinicians to better understand each other's roles, and helps prepare them to deliver better integrated care to patients and service users.

IPE is important not just pre-qualifying, where, for example, health and social care students might participate in joint scenario-based learning days, but also post-qualifying, where IPE has been shown to affect organisational behaviour and provide benefits to practice.

20.2 How to get started with professional development in an MDT

- **Identify your interests and goals:** reflect on your career ambitions or skills you'd like to improve.
- **Local opportunities:** check with your employer or NHS Trust for available training sessions, workshops or funded courses.
- **Online learning resources:** highlight widely accessible platforms such as e-Learning for Healthcare (eLfH), NHS Learning Hub, or professional association websites.
- **Networking / collaboration:** engage with peers, attend events, or join professional networks to share experiences and discover new opportunities.

Add any development opportunities that might be of interest to you below:

_____

_____

_____

_____

_____

Scenarios for guided reflection and action planning

Guided reflection is a structured process for critically analysing experiences to gain insights. It involves evaluating scenarios and outcomes for goal alignment.

Encouraging health and social care professionals to review practices in this way allows for tailored strategies for patient-centred care. This helps to develop team rapport through open dialogue and shared learning, improving reasoning and clinical outcomes.

Action planning is the process of setting achievable goals and creating actionable plans to track progress. This method builds a feedback loop, encouraging continuous development and motivating healthcare professionals to improve their practice.

By reviewing practices and setting tailored goals, we enhance patient-centred care and foster better communication within the MDT. This reflective approach builds team rapport, promotes shared learning, and improves both clinical reasoning and outcomes. Journalling is an excellent tool for emotional resilience, aiding in stress management and promoting continuous learning.

Workshops on reflective writing techniques and team debriefs help professionals develop these habits. Reflective discussions, steered by structured prompts, encourage open dialogue and allow for shared insights. Developing a repository of reflective questions tailored to health and social care scenarios can improve team cohesion and clinical excellence.

21.1 Common scenarios

Here we explore common scenarios, their implications, and actionable strategies with an MDT focus to guide your reflections at different points in the situation.

Miscommunication impacting patients' cultural needs

Cultural competence is essential for equitable healthcare delivery, fostering trust and engagement. For example, a patient fasting for religious reasons may require input from a dietitian and pharmacist to ensure nutritional and medication needs are met without compromising their faith. Without this MDT input their cultural needs may be unmet.

Addressing the issues for such a patient requires analysing potential contributing factors to poor MDT working, such as unclear roles, environmental distractions or hierarchical barriers. Equally important is a culture of psychological safety, enabling team members to speak up without fear of blame.

- Preventive actions: resolve communication breakdowns through regular team huddles, defining clear roles and responsibilities. Standardise communication frameworks to improve handovers and briefings. Conduct cultural competence training for all MDT members and develop protocols to identify and address patients' cultural needs proactively. Advocate for interpreter services or cultural liaisons and identify gaps in service provision.

Reflect on what other actions you could take with the MDT in this situation:

_____
_____
_____

A healthcare professional struggles with workplace stress, affecting their wellbeing and productivity

Burnout among healthcare workers has far-reaching implications for patient care and team dynamics.

Collective efforts such as peer mentoring, shared decision-making and flexible rostering develop a culture of mutual respect and resilience. Debriefs after challenging cases allow members to process emotions and share coping strategies. Occupational health services and wellbeing initiatives, such as mindfulness sessions or exercise programmes, provide additional support.

- Preventable actions: establish peer support programmes to facilitate open discussion about work–life balance, and utilise external resources such as employee assistance programmes for professional counselling.

A clinical error occurs requiring safeguarding of the patient

Reflect on the potential impact an error of this nature may have on the patient and MDT involved:

_____

_____

_____

While errors are inevitable in complex health and social care systems, they provide valuable opportunities for improvement.

MDT debriefs support open, non-punitive discussions, focusing on system-wide issues rather than individual blame.

Root cause analysis (RCA) helps identify gaps in training, protocols or resource allocation. For example, a medication error may highlight the need for better electronic prescribing systems or increased pharmacist involvement during ward rounds.

Transparent communication with those affected is equally important, demonstrating accountability and a commitment to learning.

- Actions: conduct RCA involving all relevant members to ensure comprehensive learning and implement changes such as updated protocols or training sessions to encourage openness in the reporting and discussion of errors.

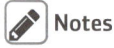 Notes

Root cause analysis (RCA) 'Five Whys' method

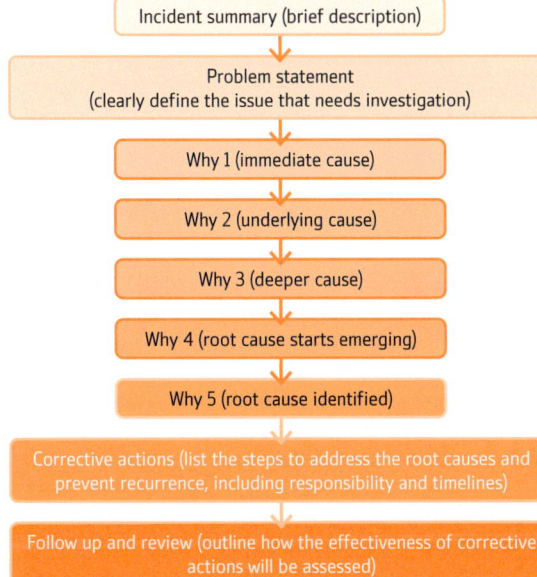

Root cause analysis 'Five Whys' method process (NHS England, 2015).

Each challenge explored underscores the importance of MDTs and how central it is for effective problem-solving and quality care.

Open communication, mutual respect and shared accountability help healthcare teams proactively address challenges, improve outcomes and foster personal and professional growth to the benefit of all.

NHS England (2015) *Five Whys: a simple tool used to understand an adverse outcome.* Available at: bit.ly/3Yz5aap.

22 Further understanding: ethics and integrity in MDT working

Ethics and integrity are core principles in health care that guide professional behaviour and decision-making. These values have been mentioned throughout this pocket guide because they form the foundation of effective MDT working. In health and social care, ethics and integrity ensure that patient care is safe, compassionate, and delivered fairly. But what exactly do these terms mean, and how are they developed within an MDT setting?

What is ethics in health and social care?

Ethics refers to **the moral principles that govern our behaviour, helping us navigate complex situations in a way that respects the rights, dignity and wellbeing of patients.** In health and social care, ethical practice ensures that all actions, decisions and care plans are in the best interests of the patient, while balancing the needs of the MDT and wider system. The core ethical principles include the following:

- **Autonomy:** respecting a patient's right to make informed decisions about their own care
- **Beneficence:** acting in the best interests of the patient, promoting wellbeing and doing good
- **Non-maleficence:** *"First, do no harm"*; this means avoiding actions that could harm the patient
- **Justice:** ensuring fairness in the distribution of resources and equal access to care for all patients.

What is integrity in health and social care?

Integrity means **being honest, transparent and accountable in all actions and decisions.** It involves adhering to ethical principles, even when faced with challenges or temptations to act otherwise. Integrity ensures that health and social care professionals act consistently with the highest standards of honesty and professionalism, prioritising patient safety and the wellbeing of all team members. Integrity is crucial in maintaining trust and respect within the MDT and with patients.

The following elements have all been reinforced already within this guide; here we explain further how they link to ethics and integrity.

- **Education and training:** ethical frameworks and integrity are taught during professional training and are reinforced through ongoing education. Regular workshops, discussions and case studies on ethical issues help team members develop a shared understanding of what constitutes ethical behaviour and integrity in the context of patient care.
- **Self-reflection:** professionals are encouraged to regularly reflect on their own values and decisions. Self-awareness helps individuals recognise any biases or shortcomings in their approach and makes them more attuned to the ethical implications of their actions.
- **Team culture:** a team culture that prioritises open communication, respect and accountability naturally fosters ethical behaviour and integrity. Encouraging honesty, mutual respect and support within the team allows ethical practices to become the norm.
- **Leadership and role models:** senior team members and leaders play an essential role in modelling ethical behaviour and integrity. Leading by example, they create an environment where ethical dilemmas are discussed openly and honestly, and where integrity is valued.

- **Learning from experience:** ethical decision-making and integrity are often shaped through real-world experiences. Professionals learn how to approach difficult situations through exposure to various patient care scenarios, peer discussions and mentorship. Over time, experience sharpens one's ability to act ethically and maintain integrity in complex situations.

> Scenario: Ethical dilemma – a patient's refusal of treatment
>
> A 65-year-old patient is diagnosed with a life-threatening condition and is advised to undergo surgery. However, the patient refuses, stating they do not want the surgery despite understanding the risks of not proceeding.
>
> Which ethical principles do you think are important in this scenario and why?
>
> _____
>
> _____
>
> _____
>
> In this situation, **ethics** (particularly the principle of autonomy) guides the team to respect the patient's decision, as long as the patient is fully informed about the potential consequences of their choice. Professionals must ensure that the patient understands their decision and is not acting out of fear or coercion. Integrity is also key here, as the team must be transparent about the risks and avoid pressuring the patient into making a different decision. The team should ensure that the patient's choice is documented and respected throughout their care, even if it's difficult for the team to accept.

Developing ethics and integrity: this scenario requires professionals to navigate a delicate balance between ethical principles (autonomy vs. beneficence) and integrity in being honest and transparent. Discussing this case with colleagues in an MDT meeting would help the team reflect on the best course of action.

Scenario: Integrity – a medication error

A nurse realises they have administered the wrong medication to a patient, but no adverse effects have been noticed. The nurse must decide whether to report the mistake.

Which ethical principles do you think are important in this scenario and why?

_____

_____

_____

Here, **integrity** is important. The nurse must admit the mistake, report it, and work with the MDT to ensure that the patient is not at risk and that appropriate corrective actions are taken. By doing so, the nurse upholds their professional responsibility and commitment to patient safety. Failure to report the error would compromise patient safety and violate the trust between the team and the patient.

Developing ethics and integrity: reporting medication errors openly helps to support a culture of transparency and learning, where team members feel supported rather than blamed. Over time, this approach reinforces the importance of integrity and accountability in the MDT.

23. The importance of self-care for health and social care professionals working within the MDT

As professionals, we dedicate our lives to caring for others, but we must also remember to care for ourselves. While our professional identity is a huge part of who we are, it does not define us completely. Balancing work and personal life can be difficult, especially in a fast-paced multi-professional environment where the needs of others often come first. However, neglecting our own wellbeing can lead to burnout and stress, and even impact the quality of care we provide to patients.

One way we can look after ourselves is by following the 'Six ways to wellbeing' available at bit.ly/433X0gr: **Connect**, **Be active**, **Take notice**, **Keep learning**, **Give**, and **Care for the planet.** These principles provide simple yet powerful ways to maintain our mental, emotional and physical health.

Connect: building and maintaining strong relationships with colleagues, friends and family helps us feel supported and valued. Within an MDT, good relationships make work more enjoyable and improve teamwork, ultimately leading to better patient outcomes.

Be active: finding ways to move our bodies, whether through walking, yoga, team sports or another activity, helps reduce stress, boost energy levels and improve mood. Physical activity is essential for both our mental and physical health, keeping us resilient in the face of daily challenges.

Take notice: practising mindfulness and being present in the moment help us manage stress and appreciate the positives in our work and personal lives. Recognising small wins, celebrating successes, and taking a step back to breathe can help us stay grounded.

Keep learning: we are constantly learning in our professional roles, but personal growth is just as important. Whether it's picking up a new hobby, attending a course or learning a new skill, continuous learning keeps us motivated and engaged.

Give: as health and social care professionals, giving is part of what we do every day. But giving doesn't have to be just about patient care – it can be as simple as supporting a colleague, mentoring a student, or doing a kind gesture for someone. Giving develops a sense of fulfilment and strengthens our connections with others.

Care for the planet: engage in activities that support environmental sustainability, such as recycling, conserving energy or participating in community clean-ups. Caring for the planet not only benefits the environment but also enhances personal wellbeing by encouraging a sense of purpose and connection to the world.

If we don't look after ourselves, we won't be able to give our best to our patients or our colleagues. Taking time to focus on our wellbeing isn't selfish – it's necessary. When we prioritise self-care, we become more effective, compassionate and resilient professionals.

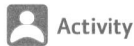 **Activity**

Six ways to wellbeing: personal reflection

This reflection table gives you space to think about your own wellbeing strategies and how you can integrate them into your daily life.

Six ways to wellbeing	What I do to achieve this	Why this is important to me
Connect		
Be active		
Take notice		
Keep learning		
Give		
Care for the planet		

Notes

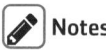 Notes